An Analysis of Medical Savings Accounts

An Analysis of Medical Savings Accounts

Do Two Wrongs Make a Right?

Mark V. Pauly

The AEI Press

Publisher for the American Enterprise Institute

WASHINGTON, D.C.

1994

ISBN 0-8447-7027-2

THE AEI PRESS
Publisher for the American Enterprise Institute
1150 17th Street, N.W., Washington, D.C. 20036

Printed in the United States of America

Contents

STANDARDS FOR COMPARISON AND JUDGMENT   3

THE MSA PROPOSAL   5

ANALYZING SOME CLOSE RELATIVES TO MSAS   6

ANALYSIS OF MSAS   9

DO ALL VERSIONS OF MSAS HAVE THIS PROPERTY?   9

STRONGER ALL-OR-NOTHING ARRANGEMENTS   15

CAN YOU SAVE MORE THAN THE DEDUCTIBLE BY BUYING
A HIGH-DEDUCTIBLE POLICY?   16

EQUITY   19

TAX CREDITS INSTEAD OF DEDUCTIBILITY   19

ALTERNATIVES TO MEDICAL SAVINGS ACCOUNTS   20

CONCLUSION   21

NOTES   23

ABOUT THE AUTHOR   25

T his book evaluates and criticizes proposals for medical savings accounts (MSAs) as devices for improving economic efficiency and equity in the medical care sector. The fundamental idea embodied in MSAs, as proposed by John Goodman and colleagues at the National Center for Policy Analysis in Dallas,[1] is to offer tax breaks for an alternative to conventional health insurance. The alternative is a tax-sheltered account that may be drawn upon for out-of-pocket medical expenditures or else saved for future spending on other things. The purpose of the accounts is to encourage individuals to purchase health insurance policies with larger deductibles than are customary under current tax law, which promotes reliance on comprehensive, low-deductible health insurance by providing an open-ended tax exclusion for purchase of employer-sponsored insurance. It is hoped that individuals will become more frugal in their use of medical services if they pay for them directly, from an account that could be converted back into cash, than if they rely wholly or partially on health insurance for those services.

Several legislative proposals in the current health reform debate in the U.S. Congress embody the MSA concept in one form or another, and additional versions with different design parameters could be fashioned. I will discuss some of the specific proposals later in this book, but at the outset I wish to consider MSAs in a more generic form. There are two key design parameters: (1) whether the account is *restricted* or *unrestricted*, and (2) whether the tax subsidy takes the form of *tax deductibility* or *tax credits*. An MSA is unrestricted if it can be created in any amount and without reference to the provisions of an individual's health insurance policy. It is restricted if it is limited to some minimum size or conditioned on an individual's purchasing a certain kind of insurance, such as a catastrophic

I am grateful to Carolyn Weaver, Eugene Steuerle, Derrick Max, and Christopher DeMuth for comments.

insurance policy, or one with a minimum deductible. Tax deductibility means that the individual can exclude MSA deposits and earnings from taxable income; the size of the tax subsidy is therefore larger for those paying higher tax rates. In contrast, tax credits subtract directly from an individual's tax liability and thereby reduce taxes at a constant rate across tax brackets. I will initially analyze the tax-deductible MSA and later consider the other variants, comparing restricted and unrestricted MSAs and finally tax credits.

I will argue that, although the MSA device has merit compared with current tax policy, it is unlikely to produce the significant improvements in the efficiency of medical care foreseen by its proponents. The policy problem, explained in detail below, is this: if the incentives to use MSAs are set at levels that will induce widespread participation, that participation will not greatly reduce and may well *increase* total medical spending. Conversely, if the incentives in MSAs are strong enough to reduce medical spending by those who use them, the proportion of the population likely to use MSAs is likely to be quite low. More fundamentally, the MSA proposal is a distraction from the basic task of health care reform, which is to present informed buyers with appropriate incentives to consider the costs and benefits of the medical care they are purchasing. Whether spending rises or falls as a result of MSAs, there is no reason to believe that the tax subsidies they provide will lead to the efficient level of spending—the level that appropriately balances the costs and benefits of medical care and medical insurance. Efficiency requires that individuals considering the purchase of medical care or medical insurance face prices that reflect the true resource costs of their decisions. If we think that service and insurance prices are close to cost, then *any* (marginal) subsidy, whether to medical services, medical insurance, or both, is inefficient, because it leads to excessive spending—to spending for services whose resource costs are greater than their health benefits.[2]

MSA proponents often characterize their proposal as a "free-enterprise," "private-market," or "individual-choice" alternative to other health care plans that rely on explicit government expenditures, employer mandates, price and spending regulation, and other forms of direct government control. This characterization draws on the common perception that encouraging private behavior by giving it a tax advantage involves less government intrusion than an outright government subsidy of that behavior. The perception is true up to a point: a heavily controlled public expenditure program is obviously different from a general, permissive tax exclusion, and there are undoubted gains in economic efficiency to be had from letting individuals choose for themselves.

Nevertheless, the extent of government control inherent in a policy is not necessarily linked to whether the policy is a direct expenditure or a tax exclusion, and the immense volume and detail of the tax code are evidence that tax inclusions and exclusions are determined with a level of legislative care comparable to direct expenditures. As we shall see, MSAs, regardless of the banner they parade under, necessarily require substantial government definition and regulation even in their most pristine academic form. As actual legislation they would undoubtedly involve even more. It is also worth noting that the fiscal consequences of tax credits, deductions, and exclusions are identical to those of equivalent public subsidies rendered under the same conditions: forgone tax revenues, like expenditures, must be offset elsewhere by higher taxes, lower spending, or an increase in the deficit. For these reasons, I will treat tax breaks as equivalent to public spending and will not hesitate to use the terms *tax subsidy* and *tax expenditure* to describe exceptions from generally applicable tax requirements made for the purpose of inducing specific private behavior.

I must emphasize, finally, that I am limiting my analysis to tax-subsidized medical savings accounts. Some firms currently offer employees the option to set aside a fraction of after-tax compensation in a medical spending account, and to return unspent funds in that account, plus interest, at the end of some period. As a superior method of budgeting out-of-pocket payments, thereby inducing individuals to take policies with lower premiums and larger deductibles, such schemes have considerable merit and may appeal to a segment of the market. For reasons I discuss later, I would expect this market to be relatively small, but it is still desirable for those who prefer it. Such unsubsidized accounts, however, funded with after-tax dollars, offer fundamentally different incentives from proposed tax-subsidized MSAs and require no special government action. It is the proposals to create government-regulated, tax-shielded accounts that are the subject of this book.

Standards for Comparison and Judgment

Two alternative comparisons can be made in evaluating health reform proposals. One standard is to compare outcomes under the proposed reform with the status quo. Since our current public policies are argued to cause medical costs to be higher than they need to be and do so in an inequitable fashion, it is usually not hard to generate a potentially better outcome. In my analysis, I will make this comparison. The other standard is to compare one reform proposal with one or more alternative proposals. In what follows, the alternative reform proposal I will consider is the major alternative free-market competitor: abolition of all tax subsidies, in particular the exclusion from taxation of premiums for employer-provided health insurance, and their replacement by tax credits. I am coauthor of one prominent version of this proposal and will describe its key features below.[3]

The objectives by which alternatives are to be judged are efficiency and equity. Efficiency has in part the obvious meaning of cost and waste minimization. It has the less obvious meaning of ensuring that the amounts and types of medical services be those for which benefits are greater than costs. One important implication of this latter meaning is that the ideal level and ideal rate of growth in expenditures are not the lowest possible; the alternative that is better, therefore, is not necessarily the one with the lower rate of growth in cost. In this sense, the question is not whether MSAs will achieve a lower rate of growth in cost than some other alternative, but whether they will achieve a rate that represents a better balancing of benefits and costs. Finding that some other policy is more likely to achieve lower costs than MSAs does not therefore imply that the alternative policy is better or more desirable. While lower rates of growth than the status quo are probably desirable, the alternative with the lower rate is not necessarily the better. The conclusion of the Congressional Budget Office,[4] for example, that MSAs "are unlikely to restrain medical spending much" is not of much value without further definition of how much is "much." The CBO should have investigated (but did not) whether MSAs will reduce costs to the appropriate level, with "appropriate" being defined as in the next section.

The efficient or appropriate level is the level at which the benefits and costs of medical services are balanced. Absent any other distortions, this balance is usually best achieved by letting consumers make decisions in markets that are both competitive and unsubsidized in any fashion. If subsidies are provided to low-income or high-risk people, they should be provided in ways that least distort the choices between medical care (or health insurance) and other goods.

Equity, or fairness, is the other standard. Unlike efficiency, equity has no rigorous, generally accepted definition. For most of this book, I will simply use the term to mean that, for people of average health, higher-income people should pay higher taxes and receive smaller subsidies than lower-income people (vertical equity), and that subsidies should be the same for people with the same income undertaking the same activities (horizontal equity). I realize that this casual usage is open to several objections. To those who believe, for example, that our current tax structure is *too* progressive from the standpoint of equity—imposing unfairly high marginal rates on higher-income taxpayers—tax deductions that disproportionately lower the tax liabilities of those in higher tax brackets, and thereby moderate total tax progressivity somewhat, may be regarded as improvements rather than defects in tax equity. My defense is that this is an analysis of a single tax proposal, not a treatise on general tax policy, and that it is conventional in such discussions—including discussions by opponents of the Clinton administration's health reform proposal who criticize it, rightly in my view, as being regressive in important respects—to take the rest of the tax structure, including its degree of progressivity, as given.

The MSA Proposal

The heart of all variants of the MSA proposal is the creation of a tax-free account from which people could pay medical bills not covered by insurance. Money deposited in the account would be deducted from taxable income, and earnings on the account would not be taxed. Some proposals, such as that of Senator Phil Gramm, permit funds to be withdrawn from the account at any time, as long as income and payroll taxes are paid; others impose additional penalties if funds are withdrawn from the account before a certain age, such as fifty-nine years. Some proposals permit the account to be rolled over, tax free, into the person's retirement fund, or used to pay for postretirement health care. Most do not. Thus there are two essential elements to the MSA approach: (1) money deposited in such accounts and then spent on medical services is excluded from federal income taxation, and (2) taxes are deferred, and in specified circumstances eventually forgiven, on deposits and earnings that are not spent on medical services. For the rest of this book I will describe MSA earnings as "interest," for simplicity. This means that the tax treatment of MSAs can be more generous than the tax treat-

5

ment of pensions or regular IRAs, in which taxes must be paid at least eventually, when money is withdrawn from the account. In the unrestricted version of MSAs, individuals are not required to purchase health insurance with a minimum-size deductible in order to have the account quality for tax breaks.

The most detailed version of a restricted approach is in the bill introduced by Reps. John Kasich and Rick Santorum, the "Health Care Savings Plan of 1992," which establishes "Medisave" accounts. These accounts are permitted when people purchase insurance policies with deductibles of at least $3,000, with a *stop-loss*, or maximum out-of-pocket cost, of $9,000. The maximum tax-free contribution to the account is $4,800; contributions can be made either directly by individuals or by employers as part of the employee's total compensation. Apparently there is no minimum contribution to the account, but the insurance policy's deductible must be at least $3,000. Senator Gramm's proposal is similar on this score. Funds withdrawn from the account before retirement would be subject to a 10 percent penalty *and* taxed as ordinary income; once the account reaches $15,000, however, excess funds could be withdrawn with no penalty except payment of income tax.

Other versions of this idea set lower limits for the amount in the MSA. Other important variables include whether the purchase of catastrophic insurance coverage is *required* in order to set up an account (for example, could an uninsured person set up an account?), and the minimum deductible that must be met if insurance is required.

Administratively, use of a debit card, administered by the entity that holds the account, is envisioned as the most convenient method of making covered medical expenditures. If a person had uninsured medical expenses in excess of the amount in the account, a line of credit, perhaps administered by the government, might be used.

Analyzing Some Close Relatives to MSAs

The easiest way to get some initial insight into what the MSA scheme would do is to compare it with alternative tax treatments of direct, uninsured medical spending. There are two critical ones: tax deductibility of all medical expenses, regardless of how financed, and flexible spending accounts. The second is currently permitted, but the first generally is not; deductibility of out-of-pocket medical expenses is currently limited to those who itemize and whose expenses exceed 7.5 percent of their adjusted gross income.

Consider for the moment a situation in which savings account interest rates are low enough to be negligible (as they are at present), in which there is no minimum or maximum contribution to an MSA, and in which there is no minimum insurance deductible to qualify an account as tax free, but in which funds withdrawn from an MSA for other consumption are taxed as ordinary income. The MSA is then equivalent to simply making out-of-pocket medical expenses tax deductible. Suppose, for instance, a family with an income of $80,000 per year has $20,000 in an ordinary bank account and purchases an insurance policy with a $3,000 deductible. Suppose the family anticipates medical bills of $2,000. If all medical expenses are tax deducted, the family saves the taxes on $2,000 worth of income and must draw its bank account down by $2,000.

Now suppose instead that the family sets up a medical savings account by taking $2,000 out of its bank account. Doing so also reduces the family's bank account by $2,000, reduces its taxes by the tax on $2,000 worth of income, and of course pays its medical expenses out of the money in its account. As long as the household can forecast its out-of-pocket payments—or as long as it can add to its account before the bills come due—there is no difference between the MSA tax break and the simpler approach of permitting all medical spending to be tax deductible.[5]

Things are more complicated if medical expenditures are unpredictable and contributions to the account must be set in advance. Contributions to the account could then be either less or greater than the actual out-of-pocket payment. If the contributions are less, the person will have to pay out of an ordinary bank account and will lose some of the potential tax savings. If contributions exceed expenses, the initial tax break is actually greater, but the fungibility of amounts deposited in the account is imperfect. The 10 percent penalty, for instance, would mean that money in the account will be slightly less liquid than money saved in a bank account. The ability to carry funds over to the next year implies that a reasonable person will not suffer much of a penalty over the long term. The family need only transfer enough from its regular account to its medical IRA to cover its maximum out-of-pocket payment. As long as the family holds positive savings account balances in excess of the insurance policy deductible, all funds to cover that deductible will eventually be run through the account and will not be subject to withdrawal penalties. A penalty would be paid only if there were a sudden demand for dissaving, or if there were some penalty when the person became eligible for Medicare and there was too much in the account. In general, however, an MSA functions as a close approximation to full tax deductibility of all uninsured medical expenses.

There is an extra advantage to an MSA relative to full tax exclusion of out-of-pocket expenses. The ability to keep account earnings free of taxation does constitute an extra break, since the earnings on earnings can accumulate tax free and can eventually be withdrawn with little or no penalty. The importance of this advantage depends on the level of the interest rate. At present, with low nominal and real interest rates, this advantage is not of much consequence. If interest rates rise, the ability to shield interest will provide a strong but distorted incentive to use MSAs.

The fundamental idea is that all uninsured medical expenses would be paid from the MSA; the deductible in the insurance plan would often equal the amount deposited in the account, and under some plans it is required to be set at this level. It is therefore incorrect to assert, as the Congressional Budget Office did in its analysis, that "the proposed coverage would expose (most people) to the risk of paying medical expenses in excess of the balances in their MSAs."[6] The risk is, rather, that the account will be wiped out. If the person initially had a policy with a $500 deductible and switched to a $2,000 deductible with an MSA of an equal amount, and if the funds for the MSA came from a virtually risk-free savings account, the net effect is that of being exposed to the loss of an additional $1,500. To be sure, the individual does increase his wealth because premiums decline, but premiums will usually decline less than the maximum increase in out-of-pocket payment. It is virtually certain, however, that he will be worse off in the worst-case, maximum-loss scenario. The reward for accepting this risk is the possibility of avoiding taxes on the *additional* tax-shielded amount—that is, on the $500 original deductible. I consider below whether this trade-off is likely to be advantageous.

There is another close parallel to MSAs. Current tax law permits employers to set up flexible spending accounts (FSAs) for their employees' uninsured medical expenses. In contrast with an MSA, these accounts do not accumulate interest for the employee; apparently the employer gets to keep any interest earned. But except for this difference, which is small at today's low interest rates, individuals who can predict their out-of-pocket payments in each year can achieve the same benefits as are available from MSAs under current tax law. In particular, the same exclusion from federal income taxation is permitted, while payroll taxes and some state and local taxes are also excluded.

The main difference between the current FSAs and MSAs occurs if the person fails to predict accurately and therefore fails to use up all the money in the account in a calendar year. In the case of an FSA, those excess funds are given to the employer instead of being rolled over into the next year's balance. At one time, a so-called zero-balance FSA did permit the individual to recover unspent funds, but that is no longer the case.

Analysis of MSAs

In the simplified, unrestricted version described above, creating tax-shielded MSAs is equivalent to offering the possibility of tax exclusion for all medical spending, whether paid nominally by employer or employee, and whether insured or uninsured. This is substantially different from the current tax treatment most Americans experience, in which payments for premiums for employer-sponsored health insurance are excluded from taxation, but out-of-pocket medical payments and insurance premiums paid by families must be paid with after-tax dollars. Restrictions that require deposit into the MSA before expenditures are incurred, or that offer additional penalties for withdrawal, reduce the tax preference slightly—especially if spending at least the amount in the account is uncertain. The primary influence, however, is similar.

Do All Versions of MSAs Have This Property?

The key issue in whether or not an MSA subsidizes out-of-pocket payments is whether the person's lifetime tax liability is affected by the level of his uninsured medical expenditures. Everyone recognizes that the MSA should not be a vehicle through which unlimited amounts of tax are avoided. Should the amount of tax be related to the level of medical spending?

Most proposals limit the amount that can be deposited tax free in the account in any one period, but they do not limit the total amount that can be accumulated. They do, however, provide for taxation and penalties if money from MSAs is used for nonmedical purposes before retirement. A few bills permit MSA funds to be rolled over without penalty or tax upon retirement. Any tax-free rollovers presumably must be accompanied by an upper limit on the amount accumulated in the account.

If money not spent on medical care is eventually taxed, while money spent on medical deductibles is untaxed, the distortion is obvious: medical care spending, whether made out of pocket or in a premium payment, is given more favorable tax treatment than other types of spending out of total compensation. That is, MSAs extend the current tax subsidy for employer-paid insurance premiums to all medical spending, whether insured or not.

For those bills that permit tax-free rollovers on retirement, the analysis of incentives is more complex. I consider two alternative possibilities: either the person deposits less than the maximum that is permitted, tax free, in his MSA, or he deposits the maximum amount every year. A person may choose not to deposit the maximum permitted tax-free amount for several reasons: he may prefer to hold savings in another taxable but less restricted form, or he may prefer taxable consumption now to tax-free savings and consumption later. In the latter case, a tax-free MSA is still equivalent to a tax subsidy of out-of-pocket payments, since such payments, in reducing the account below the desired target, offer an opportunity for further tax reductions when the account is replenished.

Suppose that the maximum tax-free annual contribution is $3,000, for example, and I wish to buy insurance with a $3,000 deductible and to hold $9,000 in this account. Suppose that the account has reached $9,000, and now I am contemplating a medical procedure that will cost more than my $3,000 deductible. Since I will then deposit $3,000 more of my income into the account to bring it back up to $9,000, the net cost to me of the procedure is reduced by the tax on $3,000.

Only in the last case, in which the person wishes to add the maximum tax-free amount to the account each period, is there no effective tax subsidy for out-of-pocket payments. Then there is no reason to believe that the individual will choose the insurance policy that best meets his demand. If, for instance, one is required to purchase a catastrophic policy with a maximum deductible specified by regulation to get a tax break, there is no reason to believe that the deductible chosen by the regulator is the one that represents the proper trade-off between risk protection and insurance premium. If incentives were neutral, I might prefer a policy with a $2,000 deductible, but I may be tempted by the tax break in Senator Gramm's bill to choose a $3,000 deductible—to take a gamble in return for a tax break. In effect, the MSA approach shares with the Clinton health bill the policy of substituting bureaucratic judgment for individual judgment—and it offers tax incentives for gambling to boot! Medical spending may fall, but people will be more unhappy.

I strongly suspect, however, that most people will not take the maximum possible deduction each year, even for those bills with tax-free rollover. Hence, it seems sensible to analyze MSAs as embodying tax subsidies to out-of-pocket spending. I will therefore interpret the effect in that fashion in what follows.

There is another way to avoid the problem of tax subsidies to out-of-pocket spending. John Goodman and Gerald Musgrave appear to propose that the amount to be deposited tax free each year in an MSA should be determined not by the employee but by the employer.[7] An employer might, for instance, make compulsory deductions of $3,000 from the amount each employee would have been paid and then deposit that amount in an MSA, at the same time compelling employees to take a policy with a $3,000 deductible. Such an approach does eliminate the distortion to individual-employee choices, because it eliminates those choices. It seems unlikely that such a forced savings plan could be viable in competitive labor markets, and in any case it represents a clear departure from an individual-choice, market-oriented approach to health reform.

Does the extension of a tax break from one type to all types of medical expense improve efficiency or equity? It is generally agreed among health economists that the current tax exclusion of employee compensation directed toward health insurance premiums is both inefficient and inequitable. It is inefficient because it stimulates excessive spending on health insurance. This in turn stimulates expenditures on medical services (because conventional insurance encourages the use of additional medical care), and it raises administrative costs in the medical care sector (because insurance payments and reimbursements involve more paperwork and other administrative costs than do direct payments for medical services). It is inequitable, because the dollar value of the exclusion is greater for higher-wage than for lower-wage workers. The effect of excluding a type of spending from taxation is to reduce the effective price of that item by the marginal tax rate. That rate can be as high as 50 percent, when federal income and payroll taxes are combined with state and local taxes; it averages 20–25 percent for full-time employees.

How would extending tax advantages to *all* medical spending, as MSAs would do, affect efficiency and equity? Making the subsidy more general will not improve equity across income classes, but it will entitle all persons in a given income class (for example, those who purchase insurance individually and those who purchase it through their employer) to receive the same tax break. That is, MSAs do not help vertical equity, but they do improve horizontal equity.

With regard to efficiency, such subsidies might improve efficiency and paradoxically lower total spending; but then, they might not. The principle behind the possible paradox is that inefficiency is caused by distorted incentives, and a more general exclusion reduces some of the distortion. They will not be as efficient, however, as eliminating all marginal medical subsidies.

Current tax policy distorts choices in the direction of purchasing more health insurance. Broadening the exclusion via an MSA reduces the distortion to insurance, but it increases the distortion toward purchasing uninsured medical care, since it places a tax subsidy on out-of-pocket dollars. It is possible, though far from certain, that the first distortion will offset the other: two wrongs *may* make a right.

To be specific, making MSAs available will probably lead some people to buy insurance with larger deductibles than would otherwise be the case. In itself, this change would appear to result in lower levels of medical spending, and this influence has been much emphasized by advocates of MSAs. But there is another, often overlooked influence. The economizing effect of a deductible of a given size is reduced when it is subsidized by a tax exclusion. In effect, MSAs induce higher levels of patient cost sharing but attenuate the strength of those higher levels. Suppose, for instance, that a person paying the marginal tax rate of 40 percent reacts to the availability of MSAs by switching from an insurance policy with a $500 deductible that is not tax shielded to a policy with an $800 deductible that is tax shielded. The net after-tax cost to him of a treatment that uses up the deductible actually *declines*, from $500 to $480 (0.6 × $800). This person will be *more* likely to seek medical care after establishing the MSA and buying the higher deductible policy. The key issue, then, is the trade-off that potential buyers will make between extending the tax subsidy to all their medical purchases and accepting the risk of greater out-of-pocket payments (net of the tax subsidy) on larger medical bills.

Consider the choice between policies with a $500 deductible and those with a $2,500 deductible. For a person who currently purchases a policy with a $500 deductible, the net tax advantage from setting up an MSA is the tax subsidy on the expected value of claims under the $500 deductible, plus any tax savings on the accumulated interest and earnings. Assume that the expected value of claims under a $500 deductible is approximately $300, while the interest on $2,500 at 3 percent per year is $75. If the person's marginal income tax rate is 28 percent, the net subsidy is thus $84 on the deductible and $21 on the interest, for a total of $105; at a 20 percent marginal rate, the subsidy totals $75. For persons who currently have access to flexible spending accounts and deposit more than $500 in those accounts, the net advantage is only the tax savings on the interest.

In return for this subsidy, the family must increase its out-of-pocket payment when an illness occurs by as much as $2,000, from $500 to $2,500. The $2,500 deductible, however, is tax subsidized, so its net cost to a family in a 28 percent bracket is $1,800, and the net *increase* in the deductible is thus $1,300 ($1,800 – $500). For lower-tax rate families, the increase in the net deductible is larger, since the tax subsidy is smaller. In return for accepting the risk of a higher deductible, the family's health insurance premium will fall.

The key variable is the value to the family of protecting itself from this increased risk. If the expected *value* of the increase in the net (after-tax) deductible is, say, $450, then a reasonable estimate of the risk premium to cover this potential loss might be as much as $125 before taxes, and $90 after taxes,[8] approximately equal to the net tax advantage of $105.

The message, then, is that there may not be substantial gains for switching to an MSA if total medical expenses are not changed by it. For low-tax rate families, an MSA is almost sure to be unattractive. For the highest-rate families, it appears to yield a small net gain (of less than $100), with the additional tax subsidy marginally offsetting the reward needed to induce the family to accept more risk.

These calculations, it should be emphasized, are highly conjectural. While the numbers chosen appear plausible, they could vary considerably—especially the risk premium. In addition, the example ignored the relative administrative costs of insurance claims payments versus those of setting up and administering an MSA. Nevertheless, the fundamental conclusion seems valid: for most Americans, MSAs do not convey substantial net financial advantages unless they can significantly affect the total level of medical spending.

What of the effect of the MSA on the level of medical expenses? At one extreme, the change in coverage raises the user price and should therefore reduce the use of medical care. Consider people who initially have policies with $500 deductibles, but then choose a higher-deductible policy with an MSA. A person in the 40 percent bracket contemplating a procedure that costs $2,500, for instance, would experience an increase in the net out-of-pocket cost, from $500 to $1,500 (or $0.6 \times \$2,500$). At the other extreme, a person in the same bracket experiencing an expense of $200 would find a *reduction* in the net out-of-pocket cost, from $200 to $120. At a 40 percent rate, user prices would fall for all expenses below $833 and rise for all expenses above that.

What would be the net impact on spending? It is difficult to say, but we do have some clues. The user charge would rise for higher-cost, more severe illnesses, where price sensitivity might be lower. Perhaps of more importance, the user charge would fall for those small-expense illnesses that seem most sensitive to out-of-pocket price.

While these estimates cannot be made precisely, they do suggest two major conclusions about MSAs shielded only from federal income taxation: (1) they are unlikely to affect many taxpayers—low-rate taxpayers will find them insufficiently rewarding, and high-rate taxpayers will find them marginally advantageous at best; (2) for those taxpayers who do choose them, the reduction in total expense is likely to be modest; there can even be an increase in total spending.

If marginal federal tax rates should be increased further, or if deposits to accounts should be shielded from federal payroll taxes and state and local wage tax, there will be an increase in the value of MSAs. The higher level of tax subsidy, however, would mean that any dampening effect on spending would be weakened.

The key point, then, is that MSAs have two effects. The first, which economists call the "cross-price" effect, encourages consumers to substitute out-of-pocket payments for insurance. Not only does this reduce administrative costs, but it also reduces the cost of care, because insurance encourages more costly care. The second effect, unfortunately, points in the opposite direction. This "own-price effect" occurs because the tax exclusion subsidizes uninsured payments—the more income people deposit and spend out of their MSAs, the lower their taxes. This feature makes deductibles and other forms of cost sharing less potent than they would be in the absence of tax shielding, and it therefore encourages more spending. Indeed, if coverage took the form of flat 20 percent coinsurance, as it often does, the availability of an MSA alternative would leave a person in the 40 percent tax bracket with two options: to insure medical expenses and pay a net of 20 percent of his cost out of pocket, or to leave him uninsured and pay a net of 60 percent out of pocket. The impact of the MSA is then to increase the net out-of-pocket payment, from 20 cents on the dollar to 60 cents on the dollar. The MSA is not quite as generous an "insurance" policy as no-deductible, conventional insurance, but it surely can be a much weaker incentive than would be obtained in the absence of tax breaks of any type.

The idea that tax-subsidized spending accounts encourage medical spending is not a new one. Indeed, the reason that the tax laws governing flexible spending accounts (FSAs) were changed in the 1980s to prohibit open-ended FSAs was precisely that open-ended (or zero-balance) accounts were thought to be too inflationary. They were then replaced by a use-it-or-lose-it provision intended to limit the inflationary effect.[9]

The experience with flexible spending accounts sheds some light on another question—if we were to set up MSAs, how many people would use them? The experience with FSAs suggests something less than a stampede. Nationally, only about 9 percent of employers, according to a recent survey, offer FSAs. Moreover, when employers make FSAs available, only a small fraction of employees use them—even though putting some money into an FSA is a virtually costless and guaranteed way to reduce taxes. At the University of Pennsylvania, for example, the largest private employer in Philadelphia, only 16 percent of eligible employees chose to set up an FSA. To be sure, an FSA offers a more constrained subsidy than would an MSA; that is why it is less inflationary. Even a small deposit, however, can offer guaranteed tax advantages, just by writing a number on a form. The low take-up rate of this MSA cousin suggests cause for concern.

Stronger All-or-Nothing Arrangements

Were there no minimum amount or minimum deductible required for an MSA, all persons paying federal income taxes would gain by starting one, ignoring administrative costs. As noted in the numerical example, covering existing deductibles does yield tax advantages— but there are no savings in insurance administration or medical costs unless the deductible is increased. Proposals for MSAs therefore often set minimum limits either to the MSA amount or to the deductible in a qualifying insurance policy. This in effect requires the consumer to make an all-or-nothing choice as to the establishment of a tax-shielded account. Such requirements will push some people into policies with higher deductibles than they would have chosen in the absence of regulation, but it will cause others to reject the MSA option. The more potent the cost-containment effects of the required minimum deductible, the lower the rate at which it will be selected. It may prove very difficult to balance these two factors to design a plan with any significant effect on costs.

Finally, suppose a restrictive MSA did lead some people to choose insurance policies with substantially higher deductibles and to reduce their total medical spending. Is this result desirable? Not necessarily. Requiring people to accept the risk associated with a large deductible in order to receive tax breaks may cause them to take *too much* risk—and the acceptance of risk is a cost to risk-averse people, whereas the subsidy payment is only a transfer from other taxpayers. The problem is not that the level of medical spending would be too low, but that the reduced spending would be achieved at the cost of too much risk.

Can You Save More Than the Deductible by Buying a High-Deductible Policy?

The arguments for the cost-saving potential of MSAs have not turned on statistical studies of the impact of subsidies on the choice of insurance or of the impact of deductibles on medical spending.[10] Instead, they have been based on examples of the premium schedules of some insurers selling individual or small-group insurance coverage, in which the premium difference between a high-deductible and a low-deductible policy is close to or exceeds the difference in deductibles. Golden Rule Insurance Company in Indianapolis, for instance, has pointed to its own premium schedule as an example of such an arrangement. Its premium for a $1,000 deductible policy in Miami is more than $1,000 lower than its premium for a $250 deductible policy.[11] The implication is that, by putting one's money into an MSA and choosing the high-deductible policy, one can be virtually guaranteed to have reduced costs.

These comparisons of premiums, however, are quite misleading. To see why, consider a simple example. Suppose the annual individual premium that an insurance company quotes for insurance with a deductible of $250 is $2,000, and suppose that this is just enough to pay the claims people make under this insurance and to allow the firm to earn a normal profit. If exactly the same population of people were to purchase a policy with a deductible of $1,000, if we ignore any effects on administrative costs, and if the use of medical services would not be changed by the imposition of the deductible, by how much would premiums change? The answer is, unless every person spent more than $1,000, the premium would fall by less than the maximum difference in out-of-pocket expenses, or $750. For people contracting illnesses that cost more than $1,000, imposition of the higher deductible would obviously save the insurer $750. But for people who would not have gotten very sick and so would not have spent as much as $750, the higher deductible obviously saves less. Indeed, for those people who would have made no claims because they used no medical care, usually about 15–20 percent of an average population, the higher deductible saves no money. Thus the average savings in claims is definitely less than $750, so the fair-return premium will fall by less than $750.

Of course, the higher deductible should discourage some people from responding to insurance coverage by seeking care and making claims; such behavior is called "moral hazard." But it should be clear that the effect of this reduction in moral hazard would have to be quite potent to generate enough savings to return $750. The assumed responsiveness of the use of care to increases in the out-of-pocket price would have to be substantially greater than what actuaries suggested to the Congressional Budget Office as reasonable premium differences.

Perhaps, however, the actuarial estimates are wrong, since some insurers actually *do* charge a premium increase for increased coverage that is bigger than the reduction in the deductible. Does this not prove that it is possible to save money? The answer is no, and the reason is that we do not know which persons buy which policy. Suppose, for instance, that the actual difference in expected claims between a full-coverage policy and a $1,000 deductible policy was $600, and suppose that an insurer decided to charge $4,400 for the $1,000 deductible policy. The insurer could cover its cost for the full-coverage policy by charging $5,000. But it could propose to charge some larger amount for the full-coverage policy. If it charged $5,800, it could then say that the difference in premiums, $1,400, was greater than the deductible.

Of course, at that premium differential, no fully informed rational person would ever buy the full-coverage policy. Some lazy shoppers, however, or people who were not informed about relative premiums might by mistake buy the full-coverage policy. So there might be some sales at that price, and there certainly could be such premium numbers in the insurer's rate book, but they would imply nothing about the difference in actual medical costs between the two plans. If the firm wished to sell both types of plan, competition would force the premium differences to approximate expected loss differences. But individual insurance firms do not target all parts of the market, and they may pay more attention to keeping their premiums more competitive for some plans than for others.

Another, perhaps less likely possibility is that the insurer does not sell any plan to any person who seeks to purchase it; instead, the company also does underwriting. In particular, it applies strict underwriting standards for purchases of its deductible plan and weaker standards for its full-coverage plan. The full-coverage plan is its plan for nonstandard risks. Then, in contrast with the previous case, it sets premiums for each plan so that each one breaks even. The premium difference could exceed the deductible, but that would be because different kinds of people, with different expected medical expenses, would be buying different plans. For the typical high-risk person who bought the full-coverage plan, switching to the deductible plan and paying so much less in premiums would not be an option, because the underwriting would not allow it.

Alternatively, we can assume uniform (but imperfect) underwriting standards and adverse selection by consumers. If only those people who expect high medical expenses were to choose the low-deductible plan, and if healthier people were to choose the high-deductible plan, and if each plan's premium were set in proportion to expected losses, then the difference in premium could greatly exceed the difference in expenses under the plans for any given individual. In effect, the difference in premium reflects the sorting of risks across plans as well as any moral hazard that might occur.

One factor, however, explains why the differential might exist and persist in the current environment, even under conditions of perfect competition and perfectly rational consumers: this is the tax subsidy itself. Suppose the premium difference for an additional $1,000 in deductibility was larger than the additional deductible—say, $1,100. With no tax subsidy, it would be wholly irrational to pay $1,100 more in premiums for $1,000 in coverage. Suppose, however, that the deductible had to be paid with after-tax dollars, while the premium could be shielded from a 40 percent marginal tax rate. Then the extra $1,100 in premiums would represent a net after-tax cost of $660, while the additional coverage could be as much as $1,000 in after-tax dollars. This provides a superb example, if one is needed, of the irrational behavior that might be traced to the current tax subsidy. But the key question is whether the MSA is the best way to cure this problem.

Equity

There is a possibility that MSAs would improve the efficiency with which people spend their money on medical care. It is only a possibility, not a certainty, and the magnitude of the improvement in efficiency—and its relationship to the inefficiencies caused by the additional taxes needed to pay the tax subsidy—is unknown. For some, however, the equity aspects of MSAs could be their most troublesome feature. As with all tax deductions, the value of the deduction rises with the individual's marginal tax rate. Even if the taxes needed to replace the tax expenditures in MSAs themselves generated no inefficiency, MSAs would still be undesirable, because they distort the purchase of medical insurance and medical care. For someone who owes no income tax, an MSA is a waste of time, while those with the highest marginal tax rates, generally those with the highest taxable income, will gain the most. If the tax exclusion is financed by an increase (or the absence of a cut that would have otherwise occurred) in federal general revenue taxation, the net effect will probably be a redistribution from low-income to high-income families. This could, of course, be offset by increasing the progressivity of the tax system at the same time. Absent such an increase, however, MSAs will provide larger net benefits for high-income families, and they may therefore be judged as inequitable.

Tax Credits Instead of Deductibility

One way to address the equity problem is to use tax credits at a constant percentage rate, regardless of income, as the vehicle for subsidizing MSAs. The Nickles bill, for example, offers credits at a 25 percent rate for MSAs or insurance premiums. This approach has some substantial advantages over the deductibility strategy. It is more equitable, and it preserves neutrality between insured and uninsured expenses. It does, however, continue to subsidize medical spending: it still has an own-price effect. Making medical care appear cheaper than it really is will necessarily lead to higher-than-ideal expenses.

Alternatives to Medical Savings Accounts

The broad contours of the analysis are fairly clear: the current, narrowly targeted tax subsidy distorts behavior, and a more general subsidy embodied in MSAs might actually distort behavior less. That is, it is possible that MSAs represent an improvement over current health policy. They may also represent a better alternative to the heavily regulated, bizarrely subsidized arrangement the Clinton administration has proposed.

But is there a yet better alternative to MSAs? In a world with no political constraints, the answer is unequivocally yes: it is the closed-ended tax credit approach proposed to replace tax deductibility by Pauly et al. in *Responsible National Health Insurance*. Under this approach, *all* tax subsidies are removed and people receive closed-ended, fixed-dollar tax credits. The argument for this approach is that it removes rather than equalizes distortions in medical care purchasing, replacing a system of inefficient and inequitable subsidies with one that offers neutral marginal incentives both to insurance purchasing and to medical care purchasing. At the same time it guarantees purchase of minimum acceptable coverage and offers more equitable distribution of subsidies. The MSA's main advantage is that it can offset the worst distortions of the current narrow tax loopholes by broadening the loopholes. The closed-end tax-credit approach, by contrast, abolishes the loopholes. In this sense, it must by definition be superior both to MSAs and to any alternatives that continue to try to influence citizen behavior through the use of tax breaks.

It is important to note that this advantage is limited to the closed-ended, or fixed-dollar, tax credits proposed in *Responsible National Health Insurance* to help low-income people afford the health insurance they are required to buy. The only purpose of the credits is to transfer income so that, after paying for health insurance, low-income people have adequate amounts left to spend on other things. These credits are *not* intended to affect behavior: individuals are obliged to purchase insurance, regardless of the size of the credit.

In this sense, the *Responsible National Health Insurance* (RNHI) plan is also more efficient than the Heritage Foundation's approach, presented in the Nickles bill, which proposes an open-ended, or unrestricted, tax subsidy. The Nickles bill, for instance, offers 25 percent, 50 percent, and even 75 percent subsidies to people who spend more on their health insurance. It does offer subsidies to MSAs (not quite as generous as those in other bills), but it still subsidizes medical care relative to other goods, and it is therefore likely to perpetuate the incentives that make medical care appear cheaper than it really is.

The minimum catastrophic coverage in the RNHI plan is intended to be a minimum. People who wish to bear risk themselves—to "self-insure," in Goodman's and Musgrave's terminology—would be expected to choose the minimum coverage. The only reason to forbid even larger deductibles, to limit the opportunity for further self-insurance, is that a social judgment dictates that such high deductibles would discourage the use of highly beneficial, socially valued care. If it is considered safe to opt for larger permitted deductibles, then such a policy should be implemented.

In this connection, it is important to note that an increase in a policy's deductible reduces the level of insurance coverage (increases the level of risk), whether or not a person has as much in a savings account as the maximum out-of-pocket payment. *Individual self-insurance is not insurance,* since the net effect of a higher out-of-pocket payment, whether paid from an MSA, conventional savings, or out-of-pocket consumption, is to reduce lifetime wealth. As noted above, tax breaks for high-deductible insurance might cause more people to choose such insurance. But we would not regard such distorted purchases as "much better" than an equilibrium in which people chose their insurance with no tax subsidies of any kind. Costs could be too low (and exposure to risk too great), compared with the optimum. Buying a policy with a $3,000 deductible exposes the person to the same risk, whether the person has a $2,000 MSA or not. Accordingly, I would not agree with Goodman and Musgrave that MSAs would improve the RNHI plan.

Conclusion

The primary advantage of the MSA proposal over proposals to abolish current tax subsidies for health insurance, such as the RNHI proposal, is political. MSAs offer the possibility—not, as we have seen, the certainty—of somewhat improving efficiency in the medical care sector, without abolishing a tax exclusion cherished by the middle class. The inequities of the current tax exclusion will remain and will probably be made worse, but some of its inefficiencies might be reduced. If abolishing or capping the tax exclusion is judged politically infeasible, MSAs might be the most feasible alternative.

This is perhaps faint praise for the MSA idea, especially coming from an economist with no particular acumen in judging political feasibility. My own ideal would be a political system in which legislators could be persuaded to do what is efficient and equitable, rather than to protect the political rents that high-wage workers and unions derive from the current tax exclusion. I am certain that economists ought to devote themselves to persuasion on the first point rather than collaboration on the second. If the political process cannot tolerate a broad-based, loophole-closing strategy, even in the face of the considerable evidence of the economic damage caused by the current loopholes, then further enlarging the loopholes may be better than nothing at all. We should not imagine, however, that the MSA proposal is a simple or unproblematic compromise between the economically desirable and the politically possible. The burden of this monograph is that MSAs, far from being a substantial economic improvement, are likely to be a small improvement at best, and may even be worse than the current policy.

Notes

1. See John C. Goodman and Gerald L. Musgrave, *Patient Power: The Free Enterprise Alternative to Clinton's Health Plan* (Cato Institute 1994), chapter 5. This book is similar in appearance to, and is described as an abridgment of, an earlier book by the same authors, *Patient Power: Solving America's Health Care Crisis* (Cato Institute 1992), but the chapter presenting a detailed description of medical savings accounts is new to the 1994 version.

2. "Efficiency" here refers to the allocation of resources, not to the government's budget per se. Offering tax subsidies, as the MSA approach does, may reduce tax revenues and increase the budget deficit, but this budgetary impact is largely a matter of taxes and transfers, not of economic efficiency.

3. See Mark Pauly, Patricia Danzon, Paul Feldstein, and John Hoff, *Responsible National Health Insurance* (Washington, D.C.: AEI Press, 1992).

4. Letter of September 17, 1992, from Robert D. Reischauer, Director, Congressional Budget Office, to Congressman Fortney (Pete) Stark, Chairman, Subcommittee on Health, Committee on Ways and Means, p. 2.

5. My example assumes that MSA savings substitute dollar-for-dollar for other family savings, and thus that the MSA's tax advantages do not induce a higher total level of savings. The extent to which the tax advantages of regular individual retirement accounts induce higher rates of savings, and the extent of the economic benefits of such higher savings rates, are a matter of disagreement among economists. In this book I am considering only the effects of MSAs on efficiency and equity in the health care sector, not their possible further effects on the savings rate.

6. Reischauer, letter to Pete Stark.

7. Goodman and Musgrave, *Patient Power*, p. 18.

8. This estimate is based on a risk-aversion parameter of –.0005, which is at the high end of empirical estimates.

9. It is true that there is an incentive to spend any money in an FSA before the end of the year, but most people are so cautious they deposit small amounts they are sure to spend.

10. The RAND Health Insurance Experiment results are not directly relevant, because the experiment did not examine tax-subsidized deductibles.

11. See Goodman and Musgrave, *Patient Power*, p. 83 (figure 5–1).

About the Author

MARK V. PAULY is the Bendheim Professor and chairman of the Health Care Systems Department, and professor of insurance and public policy and management at the Wharton School at the University of Pennsylvania. From 1984 to 1989, he served as executive director of the Leonard Davis Institute of Health Economics and is now its director of research. Mr. Pauly has published extensively in the fields of health economics, public finance, and health insurance, and he is coauthor of the AEI publication *Responsible National Health Insurance.*

AEI Studies in Health Policy

Special Studies in Health Reform

AN ANALYSIS OF MEDICAL SAVINGS ACCOUNTS:
DO TWO WRONGS MAKE A RIGHT?
Mark V. Pauly

CLINTON'S SPECIALIST QUOTA—SHAKY PREMISES,
QUESTIONABLE CONSEQUENCES
David Dranove and William D. White

ECONOMIC EFFECTS OF HEALTH REFORM
C. Eugene Steuerle

THE EMPLOYMENT AND DISTRIBUTIONAL EFFECTS OF MANDATED BENEFITS
June E. O'Neill and Dave M. O'Neill

GLOBAL BUDGETS VERSUS COMPETITIVE COST-CONTROL STRATEGIES
Patricia M. Danzon

HEALTH REFORM AND PHARMACEUTICAL INNOVATION
Henry Grabowski

IS COMMUNITY RATING ESSENTIAL TO MANAGED COMPETITION?
Mark A. Hall

PUBLIC ATTITUDES ON HEALTH CARE REFORM—
ARE THE POLLS MISLEADING THE POLICY MAKERS?
Karlyn H. Bowman

UNHEALTHY ALLIANCES: BUREAUCRATS, INTEREST GROUPS, AND
POLITICIANS IN HEALTH REFORM
Henry N. Butler